Preface

It is my intention in this book to share a portion of my journey from illness to wholeness.

I am still walking out that journey.

\-

It is not my intention to pretend that mine is the only way to walk out the journey.

Rather, perhaps some part of it may help another on her journey.

\-

Each one is different.

Each one is sacred.

May each step of your journey into wholeness be blessed.

CHAPTER 1

This Is Cancer, But You Will Overcome It!

These powerful words from the Holy Spirit both jolted and comforted me early that Saturday morning as I prayed. It was about 3:30 A.M., Saturday, May 7, 1994. I had arisen at 3:00 A. M. for my morning prayers. Quietly, so as not to disturb my husband, I went into the kitchen to fix my cup of coffee and take it and my Bible to the chair where I usually prayed in our family room.

This period in my life began two days earlier, when at a women's meeting, the reminder to get a routine mammogram had been deeply impressed into my spirit. I put it aside for the rest of the day, but the next morning as I began to get ready for work, the Holy Spirit again deeply impressed me that I needed to get a mammogram. In fact, so powerful was that message that I got my Day-Timer and made a note on Monday's date to call and schedule a mammogram as soon as possible.

By Saturday morning I knew that this was a critical message from the Holy Spirit, so I settled into my chair and thought, "I'd better do a breast self-exam because the Holy Spirit is never wrong." As I felt my left breast, I found a lump and at that exact instant the Holy Spirit spoke in the most powerful way I have ever heard Him up to that date:

"This Is Cancer, But You Will Overcome It!"

Immediately I cried out, "NO!"

Then I had to apologize to Him for saying, "NO!" I did not mean to offend Him, and I said, "I'm sorry."

However, He understood.

Almost as quickly as He spoke to me, He then deeply impressed me that I needed to stand, to face, and to fight the cancer (the enemy -satan). It was my choice. I could stand and fight and live. Or, I could run and fear and die. In the next moment, He let me know that I could get sympathy. I could get pity. I could have others feel sorry for me so I could "feel good now." And I could die. Or I could receive empathy. I could speak the Word. I could confess and walk out my healing with a minimal amount of attention to any debilitations that might temporarily occur. I would live. That, too, was my choice.

He made it very clear that I would have to fight for my life (since satan's intention was to kill and destroy me). While others could and would help me, the outcome of this battle would depend on me. The Lord had provided all that I needed to be healed. Whether I used His resources and the extent to which I used them were my choice, my responsibility, and my consequences.

Suddenly all sorts of thoughts and fears began to assault me. I had to pray and read aloud from the Word to keep the fears from overcoming me.

Burt and I were scheduled to go out to dinner and dancing that night with some dear friends and I wanted to keep that date. It was to be a fun evening. As it turned out, I decided not to say anything to Burt about this until the next day.

In the meantime, I had to wait until a "decent" hour to call our doctor. By 8:30 A.M., I decided it was not too early to call him. The doctor was a friend from church, so I did not hesitate to call him at home. He told me I could go to see the on-call physician or I could wait and come in to see him on Monday morning. He comforted me by saying it was probably just a cyst, but he would see me promptly on Monday. I chose to wait until Monday.

The rest of Saturday was filled with the usual busyness of a working woman. In the early evening, we went out with our friends. I said nothing to anyone because I did not want to spoil the evening.

Sunday morning when Burt got up, I told him I needed to talk to him. I said that there might be something very serious that was happening to me and

I asked him if he would be able to walk through this with me no matter what. He said he would. And so I told him about what had happened to me up to that point.

CHAPTER 2

Verifying the Word of the Lord

The week ahead was full of work responsibilities for both Burt and me. My husband was to be out of town at meetings all week long. I was scheduled to make my monthly presentation to the mental health center's board members. My plans, however, had to be interlaced with medical appointments.

Sunday afternoon I called my boss and asked if I could come to his home to tell him what was happening. Once there, I told him and his wife that I had found the lump in my left breast, talked with the doctor, and was to have various appointments throughout the week. However, it was important to me that I be at work as much as possible. He was very supportive and encouraged me to come and go as I needed to throughout this week.

During my first appointment with my general practitioner friend, several biopsies were taken for testing. An urgent mammogram was also scheduled. The radiologist reviewed the test results and said he was 85 percent certain that the lump was malignant. The next medical appointment was with the oncologist, who was also a family friend. He helped me look at the realistic circumstances and explore options and consequences. I was quite willing to have a mastectomy, but he encouraged me to consider a lumpectomy. He told me the results were statistically similar, given my particular situation, for those who had lumpectomies and for those who had mastectomies. So that is exactly what we opted for - a lumpectomy of my left breast. He arranged the appointment with the surgeon. After his examination, the surgeon wanted to schedule the lumpectomy on that very Friday. (All these appointments had taken from Monday to Thursday of the same week.) I asked if we could wait until the following Monday, and he agreed. What the doctors did not know was that I had to be obedient to the Lord as I walked out my healing.

Because Burt was out of town, I called him and told him the results of the tests and what the doctors had recommended. I also explained to him that I needed to be obedient to the Lord; I needed to attend the Chicago meeting that Kenneth and Gloria Copeland were holding that weekend. He agreed and we made our reservations to fly to Chicago and rent a car. We did not have a place to stay when we arrived, but we believed the Lord would provide for us. After attending the Friday night meeting, we began a search for a room. The Lord did indeed provide a lovely room for us near the meeting location. We went to the Healing School the next day. Then we flew back to Scottsbluff.

On Monday, I checked into the hospital at 6:00 A.M. for outpatient surgery. When I awoke, the surgeon had removed the tumor and I was sent home. He was certain it was malignant, but the biopsy results were not finished. On Tuesday, he called and wanted me to return for a second surgery so they could be sure that I had "clean margins." On Wednesday, I checked in again at 6:00 A.M. The surgeon said the biopsy had confirmed the tumor was malignant and not only was he planning to get "clean margins," he also planned to remove as many lymph nodes as he could find.

I awoke in my room. This time my oncologist came in to tell me they had enlarged the lumpectomy to get the "clean margins" and had removed twenty-one lymph nodes. There was microscopic cancer in one lymph node so I was scheduled to have chemotherapy followed by radiation after the surgical area had healed. During the next two weeks, the drain tubes were removed and the extra lymphatic fluid that continued to accumulate was drained until it no longer accumulated.

I was blessed because all my doctors made it very clear that I could call them or see them any time that I needed to. During this process, and from this point on, I did just that.

CHAPTER 3

Spiritual Warfare

As all the natural procedures were going on, I also had to engage in battles on the spiritual plane. The Lord had initially impressed upon me that not only did satan intend to kill me, but that the battle also was for victory in spirit, soul, and body. He indicated that the victory would occur in just that order; the body would follow the soul and the soul would follow the spirit. So I had to pursue victory moving from spirit to soul first.

The battle began the Saturday night when the Lord had spoken to me initially. The first thing I was led to do was to have communion. There was a format for communion in a Methodist hymnal I had with my music materials. In order to cleanse my whole being from the sins the Holy Spirit brought to my mind, I was impressed to write them down. So as He brought my sins to my mind, I wrote them down on many pieces of paper (because there were many sins to confess). When I was finished, He led me to 1 John 1:9: "If we confess our sins, he is faithful and just to forgive us our sins, and to cleanse us from all unrighteousness."

I wrote that promise in red ink (to symbolize Jesus' shed blood) over all my lists of sins. Then I tore the lists up into small pieces, put them in the fireplace and burned them. These two symbolic actions were to help me fight satan's accusations about the sins that I had confessed. If he accused me of them after the communion, I could respond to him that all those sins were gone, under the blood of Jesus and the Word of God. As it turned out, I was led to make a list of sins that the Holy Spirit brought to mind daily and then, in red ink, write the promise from 1 John 1:9 out over the entire list. After the first time, I was to tear up the list and throw it away.

This process of daily confession continues to this day. After five years, I was able to keep what I call "a short list" and confess my sins during my communion without needing to actually do the symbolic actions to reinforce God's truth and to help me do the necessary spiritual warfare.

On that first night following my confession of sins, I used the communion "elements" I could find (bread and water) and had communion. Then I walked and prayed for hours.

CHAPTER 4

Forgiveness

Not only was it critical that I received God's forgiveness for my sins, and thus I made daily communion part of my healing process, but it also was important to my wholeness that I forgave each one the Holy Spirit brought before me. The importance of my forgiving them was literally part of The Lord's Prayer. "Forgive us (me Phyllis) our (my) debts as we (I Phyllis) forgive our (my) debtors (those who have sinned against me)" (Matthew 6:12).

The other scripture the Lord brought to mind was Mark 11:25-26: "And when ye stand praying, forgive, if ye have ought against any: that your Father also which is in heaven may forgive you your trespasses. But if ye do not forgive, neither will your Father which is in heaven forgive you your trespasses."

A significant component of the process of forgiveness was that I ask for forgiveness from all those the Holy Spirit brought to my mind, unless by bringing up the incident it would prove hurtful to the other individual. So I wrote letters to each person who came to mind if he or she lived apart from me. If the person lived nearby, and I could, I asked them personally for their forgiveness in specific circumstances or for specific incidents.

The Lord made it very clear to me that "my business" was to be obedient to Him. It was "not my business" how or even whether those I asked for their forgiveness responded to me. That was between Him and each of them. The goal was to cleanse me and make me whole - spirit, soul, and body. There was to be no entry point for satan to attack me. And there was to be no static in the ambience around me that would hinder healing.

A significant part of the process of forgiving was for me to forgive myself. That process became part of my healing. If God forgave me, I must forgive myself, too. In my spiritual journey up to this time in my life, I had learned to substitute the names of people I was praying for into the scripture I was using in their behalf. So it was time for me to do that in my own behalf.

I got my Bible and began to find all the healing scriptures I knew and could find in the concordance. As I found them, I began to make a list of them while writing out each one completely with my name inserted in the appropriate spot. The list was long and kept growing. At night before I went to bed, I read aloud what I had written. Hearing the Word spoken by me about me was powerful to my soul. What was made important to me by the Holy Spirit was that I had whatever I confessed. So confessing healing was critical to manifested healing.

At the Kenneth Copeland conference, I got more books and tapes about healing and began to read and apply them. (A list of books and tapes that helped me appears in the bibliography.)

During the time before any physical procedures took place, I was impressed that what Burt said was just as important as what I said. We agreed to make positive confessions to all others when asked, "How's Phyllis?" We found several truthful, positive answers to use. They proved to be invaluable. Not only did I want the positive power of God's Word working deeply in me - in every cell - but I also wanted only positive comments in the ambience surrounding me. Negative talk about me was like static in the air and only made the positive journey harder. Some of the phrases that were helpful were:

"She's doing just fine, thanks."

"She's doing better, thanks."

"I'm perking right along."

"I'm doing just fine, thanks."

And of course, "By the stripes of Jesus I'm healed."

When I went in for tests following all the procedures, I told the techs, the doctors, and whoever was there: "I am going to have a good report."

At first, they would say, "We certainly hope so," or "Well, we'll just wait and see, won't we?"

But time after time as I went in and made these positive confessions and they proved to be true, those I made the statements to began to respond, "Yes, you will, Phyllis," or "That's right, Phyllis."

At work I confessed, "By the stripes of Jesus I'm healed." So much that people quit asking me how I was. One woman in a service club I belonged to said, "I'm confused, Phyllis. They say you have cancer, but you say you're healed." And it was true.

In addition to writing down the scriptures with my name in each, I also wrote down statements to various parts of my body. I talked to my body: to my cells, to my veins, to my arteries, to my muscles, to my nerves, to my blood, to my lymph nodes, to my lymphatic fluid, to whatever parts the Lord led me to speak to. This speaking confession was part of my bedtime routine for at least five years or more. My body knows my voice and it responds to my confession quicker and more powerfully than to anyone else's voice.

Eventually, the list of scriptures and confessions got so long that I was awake a long time before bed just to confess them aloud. I wondered how to make this process more helpful to me. Then the Lord led me to put all these confessions on tape. It took two 90-minute tapes to complete. I used all of one tape and half of a second audio tape to record my confessions to me: spirit, soul, and body. Then I added these tapes to the "Healing Praise" tape from the Kenneth Copeland Ministries' series. I used a headset with my tape recorder and listened to these tapes on automatic rewind all night long. I always slept well. I learned to change the batteries as needed or the tapes in the dark. And I never kept my husband awake as I received this portion of my healing prescription.

In fact, at the second or third chemotherapy session, my oncologist said, "Phyllis, it seems like your body is working with us."

I answered, "Of course it is. I'm talking to my veins, arteries, and cells. I'm talking to my body and telling it that it must work with the treatments."

Fear was a major enemy used by satan, so I had to find scriptures to confess to bring victory over fear. Sometimes my mind would race with thoughts of fear and "what-ifs" as I was getting ready to go to work. Often I had to look at myself in the mirror and say aloud, "Thoughts, you line up with the Word of God."

In all, I had two surgeries (lumpectomies), six months of chemotherapy and thirty-four radiation treatments. I had a wonderful boss and I continued to work throughout the chemotherapy and radiation treatments. I did not experience nausea (except once after I drank apple juice instead of orange juice after a chemotherapy treatment). I did not lose my hair. I did not get burned from the radiation treatments.

However, I did get tired toward the end of each major portion of the treatment process.

CHAPTER 5

Food and Nutrition

Nutrition and supplements also became a battlefront for my victory. Just like other components of the healing process, this routine is what I did. It is not what anyone else "should" do. It is only offered as a report of my journey. Each person must make her own choices along the way.

Initially, I began to use Essiac Tea as regularly each day as if it were a medicine. In fact, I considered it as part of my own personal "prescription" for healing. I took three doses of 2 oz. each daily. Then I lowered the number of times I took it to once in the morning and once at night. When we traveled, I carried the tea with me, just like my vitamins and other medications.

Routinely my meals were all the same as indicated below unless for some specific reason I had to change them. Breakfast included one banana, one-half cup of All Bran, and one-half cup of cottage cheese. Lunch was one can of tuna in spring water and one orange or one apple. Dinner was one-half cup (or more) of broccoli, one-half cup cabbage (or more), and one orange or one-half cantaloupe. When I had to modify the meals in public, I came home and compensated by eating what I needed to finish that protocol.

In addition to this nutrition, I began to supplement the food with vitamins and minerals. These included Beta Carotene, Vitamin E, Vitamin B, Vitamin C, Calcium, Zinc, Magnesium, and Iron. I also took my prescribed thyroid medication and my chemotherapy treatment, Tamoxifen. I rotated vitamins for the morning every three days. The rest stayed the same at lunch and at dinner.

I still take vitamins, but the strength of each and the routine I follow have been modified over the years as I am led.

Of course, I followed each of my doctors' sets of instructions. I took my medication as it was prescribed. I checked with my oncologist about the various additions to my wellness routines. In cases when he told me not to use an item, I did not. But when he indicated that the item (for example, the tea) would be helpful, I included it. Thus, in all the expected positive processes that were occurring, I was in harmony with those the Lord had brought to me.

At one critical decision point, two of my doctors disagreed about the best alternative for my next step. The radiation oncologist and my other oncologist did not agree about the total area to receive radiation treatments. After each one had separately told me what he thought was my best alternative, they also told me it was my decision to make. I had one weekend to decide. The treatments were scheduled. The preliminary simulation and tattooing were completed. I agreed to let the radiation oncologist know my decision so the final calculations could be completed before I went for the first treatment.

My source of all wisdom and knowledge was the Lord. My prayer partners had been with me from the beginning, so I called them. I was led to go to the third doctor, the surgeon, to help me make this decision. My prayer partners agreed with me that the Lord would give him the "right" answer. So I called and scheduled an appointment with him at 7:00 A.M. on the Monday I was to give the radiation oncologist my answer. The caveat was, I was not to tell the surgeon that he was receiving and giving me the Lord's answer.

So, at 7:00 A.M. we met. I told him the alternatives set before me and asked him which he would suggest. As first, he would not pick one-- perhaps not wanting to be perceived as choosing one fellow medical doctor's recommendation over the other. But I asked him, "If I were your wife, what would you tell me to do?"

He then selected one alternative and told me his reasoning. I thanked him and left. Immediately I went to the radiation oncologist and told him my decision. With one of his staff members present, I told him I would absolve him of any malpractice concerns that might arise later. (The alternative I wanted was not his selection.) After that, we began the radiation treatments.

About two months after I had finished the treatments, my oncologist asked if the radiation oncologist had given me his message. He had not. As it turned out, my oncologist had gone to special cancer education meetings in California and during one session of questions and answers, he had asked the expert presenter about my situation and my choices. He asked the expert which was the better alternative. The expert said that the one I had selected was the best for me.

What joy to get confirmation that the Lord was guiding all of us! Eventually, I told my surgeon what I had done.

CHAPTER 6

Why, Lord?

One of the persistent questions early in the journey was, "Why, Lord? Why me, Lord?"

As I sought to find an answer, He led me to the answer at several levels of my being.

At the deepest level, He showed me that He promised to give us "the desires of (our) heart" (Psalm 37:4). Burt's father passed away in August 1984 and my mother in November 1984. Then my father passed away in September 1986 and Burt's mother in March 1990.

Before his death in one of his angry and difficult times, my father had said, "Now that Mom's dead, there's no one alive who loves you."

Because I was so numb from sorrow and so tired from taking care of him, I did not question what my father said.

These angry words would stay with me - festering - and ultimately they became part of what I believed as "truth." So after several years, I believed deep in my heart that since there was no one alive who genuinely loved me anymore, the best thing for me to do was to die. Thus, my body began to give me "the desire of my heart" - that I should die.

At another level, He made clear to me that to ask "Why me?" was to be answered with "Why not me?" After all, there were many people who were being diagnosed with cancer. "Time and chance happeneth to them all" (Ecclesiastes 9:11). It was just as reasonable to have it be me as to have it not be me.

At the most public level - one that I could easily share with others - He said, "It's a waste of your energy to struggle with a 'why' question. You need all your energy to fight to be whole. Don't dissipate your energy by dealing with 'why.'"

As a result of these insights from God's Holy Spirit, I stopped dealing with the question of "why."

I did, however, have to dislodge the lie from satan, via my father's angry comment, that there was no one alive anymore who loved me. The healing of this would come about through the process of forgiveness and communion that the Lord had given to me at the beginning of my journey.

<u>Epilogue</u>

The original 2008 publication of *This is Cancer, But You Will Overcome It!* closed with the declaration "It was cancer, but I have overcome it."

This was true for over twenty years, but in the autumn of 2015, my grandmother, Phyllis, was diagnosed with a recurrence (metastasis) of breast cancer. As a child, I was generally aware of my grandmother Phyllis' past battle with breast cancer, but since I was only three years old at the time of her initial diagnosis, it seemed more like a distant memory than the life-changing journey so often described by cancer patients. However, I was intimately involved in the second chapter of her breast cancer fight.

At some point, I decided that I wanted to re-publish her book, in order to honor her spirit and positivity, as well as to provide a resource for the cancer patients of today. My grandmother's priority (in regards to her book) has always been to reach the most people. As a family, we discussed whether or not it would be appropriate to re-publish her book, considering this is a cancer battle that she did not win.

Ultimately we elected to keep the original content, unchanged, with the exception of the updates in this epilogue. We desired to maintain the spirit and message of the original book. In our eyes, she did indeed overcome cancer.

For over twenty years since her initial diagnosis of breast cancer, my grandmother lived a fruitful, loving, productive, and most importantly, cancer-free life. She moved halfway across the country to be nearer her family and grandchildren, composed a symphony, wrote hymns, and regularly played the organ. She was surrounded by a loving family, including her husband (Burt), daughter, son-in-law, and two grandchildren.

If this book finds you beginning your own cancer journey, my wish for you is to discover your own message of hope somewhere in these pages. I hope the reader understands the underlying theme that each cancer patient and his or her story is unique. This was my grandmother's story. And while cancer ultimately took her life, the diagnosis of cancer all those years ago was not the end. It was indeed cancer, but she overcame it for nearly 25 years.

Sincerely

Blake Oliaro
Grandson of Phyllis Weichenthal

August 2018

My Confessions

Here are some of the Word-based confessions that I believed and spoke aloud daily:

I (your name) am the righteousness of God in Christ (2 Corinthians 5:21).

-

I (your name) am a joint-heir with Christ (Romans 8:17).

-

I (your name) am a child of God (Romans 8:16).

-

God always causes me (your name) to triumph in the Anointed One, the Lord Jesus Christ (2 Corinthians 2:14).

-

Christ has redeemed me (your name) from the curse of the law, that the blessing of Abraham might come on me (your name) through Jesus Christ. 1 (your name) receive the promise of the Spirit through faith (Galatians 3:13-14).

-

1 (your name) am Abraham's seed and an heir according to the promise because 1 (your name) am Christ's (Galatians 3:29).

-

1 (your name) am called unto liberty. 1 (your name) use that liberty to serve others with God's love (Galatians 5: 13).

-

1 (your name) am led by the Spirit of God, and 1 (your name) am not under the law (Galatians 5: 18).

-

Because I (your name) am sowing to the Spirit, I (your name) am reaping life everlasting (Galatians 6:8).

-

In Christ Jesus, I (your name) am a new creature (Galatians 6:15).

-

I (your name) am a sweet savor of Christ unto God, both to those who are saved and to those who are not yet saved (2 Corinthians 2:15).

-

I (your name) am a partaker of the inheritance of the saints in light. God has delivered me (your name) from the power of darkness and has translated me (your name) into the kingdom of His dear Son, the Son of His love (Colossians 1:12-13).

-

Jesus was wounded for my (your name) transgressions and bruised for my (your name) iniquities. He took the punishment for my (your name) peace upon Himself, and by His stripes I (your name) am healed (Isaiah 53:5).

-

Jesus bore my (your name) sins in His own body on the tree of Calvary so that I (your name), now dead to sin, can live unto righteousness. By the stripes of Jesus I (your name) was healed (1 Peter 2:24).

-

I (your name) am overcoming the devil by the precious, holy, powerful shed blood of the Lamb and by the word of my (your name) testimony (Revelation 1 2:11).

-

All the promises of God in Christ for me (your name) are yea and Amen unto the glory of God (2 Corinthians 1:20).

-

I (your name) am an anointed member of the Body of Christ in the earth (2 Corinthians 1:21).

-

God is not a man that He should lie. What He has spoken in His Word and by His Spirit to me (your name) He will do (Numbers 23:19).

-

God's Word will not return unto Him void, but it will accomplish in me (your name) that which He pleases and it will prosper in the thing(s) whereto He sends it (Isaiah 55:11).

-

God is a rewarder of me (your name), because I (your name) diligently seek Him (Hebrews 11:6).

-

God is the Lord who heals me (your name) (Exodus 15:26).

-

I (your name) am a member of Jesus' flesh and of His bones (Ephesians 5:30).

-

For God has not given me (your name) the spirit of fear, but of power, and of love, and of a sound mind (2 Timothy 1:7).

-

The Lord is the strength of my (your name) life; of whom shall I (your name) be afraid? (Psalm 27:1).

-

Let the weak say, I (your name) am strong (Joel 3:10).

-

I (your name) can do all things through Christ who strengthens me (your name) (Philippians 4:13).

-

He who began a good work in me (your name) will perform it until the day of Jesus Christ (Philippians 1:6).

-

Greater is He who is in me (your name) than he who is in the world (1 John 4:4).

-

I (your name) am more than a conqueror through Christ who loves me (your name) (Romans 8:37).

-

Bless the Lord, o my soul; and all that is within me (your name), bless His holy name. Bless the Lord, o my soul, and forget not all His benefits: Who forgives all my (your name) iniquities, Who heals all my (your name) diseases; who redeems my (your name) life from destruction; Who crowns me (your name) with loving kindness and tender mercies; who satisfies my (your name) mouth with good things; so that my (your name) youth is renewed like the eagle's (Psalm 103:1-5).

-

Then I (your name) cry unto the Lord in my (your name) trouble, and He saves me (your name) out of my(your name) distresses. He sent His Word and healed me (your name) and delivered me (your name) from all destruction (Psalm 107:19-20).

-

I (your name) will not fear, for God is with me (your name); I (your name) will not be dismayed, for He is my (your name) God; He will strengthen me (your name); yea, He will help me (your name); He will uphold me (your name) with the right hand of His righteousness (Isaiah 41:10).

-

I (your name) will not Fear, for God has redeemed me (your name), He has called me (your name) by my name (your name); I (your name) am His. When I (your name) pass through the waters, He will be with me (your name); and through the rivers, they will not overflow me (your name); when I (your name) walk through the fire, I (your name) will not be burned; neither will the flame kindle upon me (your name) (Isaiah 43:1-2).

-

As I (your name) serve the Lord, He will bless my (your name) bread and water, and He will take sickness away from the midst of me (your name) (Exodus 23:25).

BIBLIOGRAPHY

Capps, Charles. *God's Creative Power for Healing*, Harrison House, Inc., Tulsa, Oklahoma, 1991.

Copeland, Kenneth and Gloria. *Healing Praise*, KCP Records, Inc., Newark, Texas, 1991.

Copeland, Kenneth and Gloria. *Healing Promises*, Harrison House, Inc, Tulsa, Oklahoma, 1994.

Copeland, Kenneth. *How to Receive Communion*, Kenneth Copeland Publications, Fort Worth, Texas, 1992.

The Holy Bible. The Authorized King James Version, The World Publishing Company, Cleveland, Ohio, 1945.

The Methodist Hymnal. *The Methodist Publishing House*, Nashville, Tennessee, 1966.

Osteen, Dodie. *Healed of Cancer*, Lakewood Church Publication, Houston, Texas, 1986.

ABOUT THE AUTHOR

Phyllis B. Weichenthal was born in Imperial, Nebraska. She has a B.A. from the University of Nebraska-Lincoln (1959); a M.A. from South Dakota State University (1962); and a Ph.D. from the University of Illinois-Urbana (1980). In 2000, she retired from a mental health center where she had regional oversight for the substance abuse treatment services offered in the thirteen counties of the Nebraska panhandle. Phyllis started playing the piano at age four. At age seven, she began playing for the United Methodist Church and has been organist/pianist for various denominations since that time. At age thirteen, she accompanied her hometown community choir as organist in their performance of Handel's Messiah. She was the organist/pianist for the First United Methodist Church in Loomis, California. She has composed a symphony as well as a recording of various piano classics. Phyllis and Burt, her husband of fifty-eight years, moved to Granite Bay, California, in 2000 to be near their family. They have a daughter (Susan), a son-in-law (Jerry), a grandson (Blake), a granddaughter (Tessa), and two fluffy, white, Maltese dogs (Benji and Candi).

Made in the USA
Lexington, KY
12 May 2019